CLINICAL LACTATION
A Visual Guide

Kathleen G. Auerbach, PhD, IBCLC

Jan Riordan, EdD, FAAN, IBCLC

Jones and Bartlett Publishers

Sudbury, Massachusetts

BOSTON   TORONTO   LONDON   SINGAPORE

World Headquarters
Jones and Bartlett Publishers
40 Tall Pine Drive
Sudbury, MA 01776
978-443-5000
Info@jbpub.com
www.jbpub.com

Jones and Bartlett Publishers Canada
2100 Bloor Street West, Suite 6-272
Toronto, ON M6S 5A5
CANADA

Jones and Bartlett International
Barb House, Barb Mews
London W6 7PA
UK

Production Credits
Senior Acquisitions Editor: Greg Vis
Production Editor: Linda DeBruyn
Manufacturing Buyer: Therese Bräuer
Production Service: Clarinda Publication Services
Composition: The Clarinda Company
Printer: Quebecor-Kingsport
Cover Design: Dick Hannus
Cover Photo: Kathy Herbers

Library of Congress Cataloging-in-Publication Data

Auerbach, Kathleen G.
    Clinical lactation : a visual guide / Kathleen G. Auerbach and
Jan Riordan.
    p. cm.
   Includes index.
   ISBN 0-7637-0919-0
   1. Lactation Atlases.   2. Breast feeding—Complications Atlases.
I. Riordan, Jan.   II. Title.
   RJ216 .A94 1999

                             99-28577
                             CIP

Printed in the United States of America.
04 03 02   10 9 8 7 6 5 4 3

CONTENTS

Acknowledgments   vii

Foreword   ix

Foreword   xi

Introduction   1

1 Breast/Nipple Variations   3

1.1   Breasts   4

1.2   Nipples   8

    1.2.1 Size   8

    1.2.2 Dimpled Nipples   12

    1.2.3 Bifurcated Nipples   12

    1.2.4 Folded Nipples   12

    1.2.5 Double Nipples   14

    1.2.6 Inverted Nipples   16

Critical Thinking Activities   19

2 Conditions Affecting the Nipples and/or Breasts   21

2.1   Psoriasis   22

2.2   Poison Ivy   24

2.3   Allergy to Antifungal Cream   24

2.4   Impetigo   26

2.5   Dermatitis   26

2.6   Burns from Garlic (Home Remedy) Treatment   26

2.7   Candidiasis of the Nipples   28

2.8   Raynaud's Phenomenon of the Nipple   34

2.9   Accessory/Supernumerary Nipple Tissue   36

2.10 Breast Engorgement   40

2.11 Breast and Nipple Trauma   42

2.12 Mastitis   46

2.13 Galactocele   46

2.14 Abscess   48

2.15 Scarring of the Breast   52

2.16 Breast Asymmetry and Hypoplasia   58

Critical Thinking Activities   63

3

Infant Conditions   67

3.1   Buccal Fat Pads in a Normal Infant   68

3.2   Hemangioma of the Tongue   68

3.3   Cleft of the Lip and/or Palate   70

3.4   Ankyloglossia (Tongue-Tie)   72

3.5   Thrush in the Infant   74
      3.5.1 Oral   74

      3.5.2 Diaper Area   74

Critical Thinking Activities   77

Answer Key   79

Index   81

ACKNOWLEDGMENTS

No book, particularly one with a clinical orientation, is the product of its authors alone. Our colleagues impressed us with the need for a collection of photographs relating to lactation and were the guiding force behind our effort. Many clinicians enthusiastically contributed photographs. They are named below and represent leadership in the lactation field. We salute them.

- Tanna Case-Taylor (Yakima, Washington USA)

- Michael Cooney/Naturist Society (Oshkosh, Wisconsin USA)

- Robin Egbert (Cincinnati, Ohio USA)

- Karen Foard (State College, Pennsylvania USA)

- Catherine Watson Genna (Woodhaven, New York USA)

- Kathy Herbers (Naperville, Illinois USA)

- Kay Hoover (Morton, Pennsylvania USA)

- Kathleen Huggins (San Luis Obispo, California USA)

- Chele Marmet/Lactation Institute (Los Angeles, California USA)

- Lana Matthews (Ottawa, CANADA)

- Carolyn Lawlor-Smith, Laureen Lawlor-Smith, and Jill Bruce (Happy Valley, South Australia AUSTRALIA)

- Jack Newman (Toronto, Ontario CANADA)

- Ellen Petok (Woodland Hills, California USA)

- Linda Stewart (San Diego, California USA)

- Diana West (Gaithersburg, Maryland USA)

- Barbara Wilson-Clay (Manchaca, Texas USA)

FOREWORD

Anthropologists tell us that breastfeeding is Nature's way, and that virtually everyone was breastfed during the course of human evolution. However, something happened on the road to the twentieth century. Refrigeration was developed, canning and bottling techniques were perfected, an alternative feeding method was introduced, and the aggressive marketing techniques of the formula manufacturers, along with other socioeconomic factors, ensured the too-ready acceptance of artificial infant food.

The development of new technologies in maternal-infant care, while improving the physical health and well-being of mothers and their babies, further interfered with their crucial mutual interactions. The creation of the central nursery system after the second World War, and the inappropriate hospital routines that it necessitated, contributed greatly to the many iatrogenic problems seen by health care workers, and to a high breastfeeding failure rate. Indeed, many of the needs of the maternal/infant dyad were largely forgotten on the formula-oriented postpartum floors after 1950, and too many new mothers, discharged uninformed, unsupported, and discouraged, reached for the bottle instead of the telephone at the first sign of breastfeeding difficulty. The incidence of mothers nursing their babies, reaching a nadir of 22% in 1972.

In the late 1970s and 80s, largely because of the rise of naturalism, feminism and the burgeoning of research underpinning the nutritional, immunological, and emotional superiority of human milk feeding, the wheel was reinvented. We are experiencing a breastfeeding renaissance that continues to gather momentum as our century draws to a close. The American Academy of Pediatrics, in its strongest policy statement ever, recommends human milk as the preferred feeding for all newborns, including premature and sick newborns (1997). The AAP recommends exclusive breastfeeding for the first six months, and nursing continuing, with the addition of supplemental foods, throughout the first year and beyond. Physicians, lactation consultants, and all other health care providers are called upon to become knowledgeable about the management of the nursing dyad and to enthusiastically promote and support breastfeeding.

An increasing number of mothers understand that human milk is the ultimate health food and are determined to nourish their new infants with this ideal form of nutrition. Those of us in the field of lactation and in the care of the newborn are obligated to constantly enlarge our clinical experience and improve and refine our diagnostic acumen and management techniques. We will be challenged daily in our professional lives by the infinite variations of normal vs. abnormal anatomy, and by the protean presentations of clinical management problems.

This excellent and much needed manual which you are about to read, is filled with photographs of the entire spectrum of common to rare conditions of the breast, nipples, and areolae, and conditions in the infant which may lead to management problems during breastfeeding. The authors offer us in this collection of photos and accompanying text a marvelous opportunity to improve our expertise in helping mothers to fulfill their goal of a successful breastfeeding experience.

Marvin S. Eiger, MD

Dr. Eiger, M.D. is the co-author of *The Complete Book of Breastfeeding* (with Sally Olds). He is Associate Clinical Professor of Pediatrics at The Mount Sinai School of Medicine, New York. Dr. Eiger is the founder and former director of the Comprehensive Lactation Program at Beth Israel Medical Center, New York. He is the Breastfeeding Coordinator of the American Academy of Pediatrics, District 3, Chapter 2, New York.

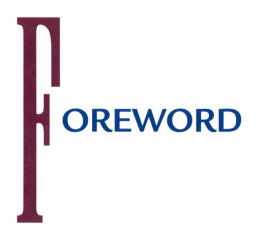

OREWORD

Where was this text when I was studying for my board exam back in 1987? Not only would it have made passing the exam much easier, but I would have been a better clinician for it. *Clinical Lactation: A Visual Guide* fills a much needed gap in reference materials for anyone either working in the field or studying to become an International Board Certified Lactation Consultant (IBCLC). Unfortunately, the available breastfeeding texts are woefully lacking in color pictures. Seeing photographs in shades of grey, while better than nothing, are not nearly as helpful as seeing a more accurate representation of an unusual condition in living color.

The slides and videos used during the lactation management course I teach are wonderful in enabling the students to picture various problems, but it is frustrating for them not to be able to go home with something to look at and study. By the end of the six day program, it is hard for them to remember which condition was which! Studying the pictures in this text will be incredibly helpful to both the students as they are garnering their breastfeeding consultancy hours, and to more experienced IBCLCs who may suddenly come across an unusual nipple problem. Now when a question comes up—is it thrush? Is it eczema? Is it a reaction to an ointment?—the consultant will have some excellent photos for comparison.

A lactation consultant is often in an isolated position of being the only one in a work setting. Usually there is no one else around to take a look and render a second opinion when something out of the ordinary presents itself. I'll be glad to have this book on my shelf when that time comes.

Jan Barger, RN, MA, IBCLC

Jan Barger is the director of the Breastfeeding Connection, a lactation consultant in private practice and with a pediatric group in the Chicago area, with many years of experience. She is a former President of ILCA.

INTRODUCTION

Lactation is coming of age as a legitimate subject for scientific investigation, clinical assessment and analysis. Thus, it is inevitable that a book of photographs of clinical situations is needed. Clinical details and physical subtleties cannot be described in words alone. If one picture is worth a thousand words, then the 104 color photographs in *Clinical Lactation: A Visual Guide* surpass volumes of written material.

This book is the result of many requests from lactation consultants in clinical practice and from students of lactation science seeking resources to enable them to identify the variety of conditions that affect the breastfeeding course. (We challenge our colleagues to join us in advancing the field by seeking permission from patients to photograph clinical situations and sharing those representations with others.)

Breastfeeding too often falls between the cracks of pediatric and obstetrical care. This book seeks to fill this gap by providing a visual story of clinical situations seen in practice. It is written for use by childbirth educators, dietitians, lactation consultants, midwives, nurses, occupational and physical therapists, physicians and other health care providers who work with breastfeeding women and infants.

Our aim is two-fold. First, we seek to highlight variations in breasts/nipples well known by professionals in clinical practice but often unrecognized by persons with less experience. Second, we include examples and cases of more complex situations that can interfere with breastfeeding.

The book is divided into three chapters. Chapter 1 illustrates the broad range of variations seen in human breasts, nipples, and areolae. Readers will note and appreciate the wide divergence of anatomical presentations of nipples and breasts. We entreat readers to guess which are which by answering the questions that accompany the photographs (answers are located at the back of the book). We wish to make the point that it is not easy to discern the maternal history of women by simple visual assessment.

Chapter 2 presents numerous conditions affecting the breast and nipples and should be of valuable assistance to the beginning practitioner. In addition to the photographs, we have included case information that will benefit clinicians in choosing appropriate treatments and interventions if they are needed.

Chapter 3 identifies infant conditions that can affect the breastfeeding experience of the newborn and subsequently the mother's lactation course.

Although we have provided information on some cases, we refer readers to our text, *Breastfeeding and Human Lactation* (second edition) for specific interventions and treatments for each condition. Any treatments and interventions used need to be individualized and based on an assessment of the total situation.

Finally, we offer the following caveat to our colleagues—lactation professionals—and readers: Most of the conditions pictured here are uncommon and are not representative of the vast majority of mothers' and babies' experiences.

1

Variations in Breasts, Nipples, and Areolae

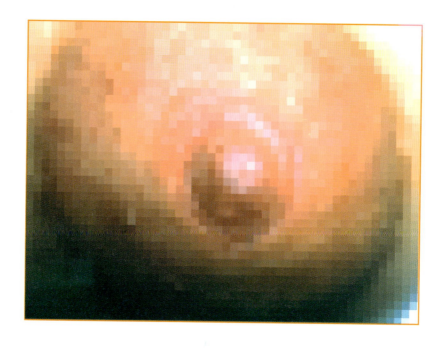

1.1 Breasts

As seen in this section, breasts come in various shapes and sizes. While normal variations usually do not affect the woman's ability to breastfeed her infant, keep in mind the relationship between form and function while viewing these photographs. Form follows function, i.e., the shapes of the breast and the infant's oral structure are a teleological "fit," meaning they have evolved over the millennia so the infant will gain sufficient nutriment to grow and thrive. Conversely, does function follow form as in the case of the large breasted mother who has difficulty feeding a tiny premature infant? And, in what cases might function alter form?

While many of the women pictured in Chapter 1 have breastfed, others have neither breastfed nor experienced pregnancy. Which is which? We invite readers to answer the questions below as a self-test of their ability to assess breasts by visual inspection alone. The answers may be found on page 79 (Note: More than one photo may answer each question).

Look at **Plates 1 through 18** and try to identify:

1. Which woman has never been pregnant?
2. Which woman is the oldest in the collection? Note: She is 61.
3. Which woman is the youngest in the collection? Note: She is 20.
4. Which woman has breastfed only one baby?
5. Many of the women in the collection have breastfed at least one child. Which woman has breastfed at least four children?
6. Which woman has breast implants?
7. Which woman has had breast reduction?
8. Which woman is Hispanic?
9. Which woman has had surgery to remove breast cysts and/or benign tumors?

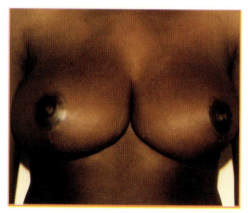

PLATE 1. *(With permission, Kathleen Huggins)*

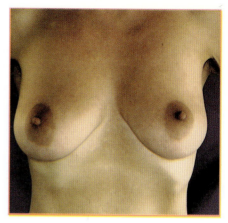

PLATE 2. *(With permission, Michael Cooney/Naturist Society)*

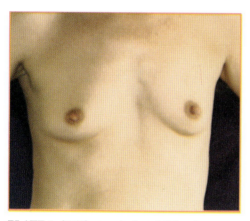

PLATE 3. *(With permission, Michael Cooney/Naturist Society)*

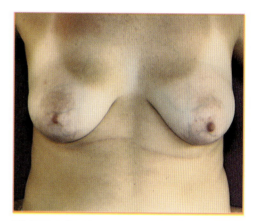

PLATE 4. *(With permission, Michael Cooney/Naturist Society)*

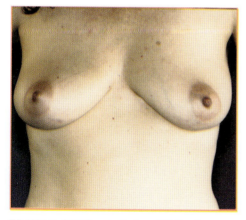

PLATE 5. *(With permission, Michael Cooney/Naturist Society)*

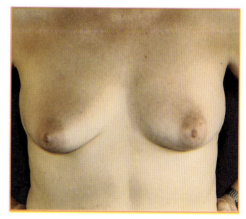

PLATE 6. *(With permission, Michael Cooney/Naturist Society)*

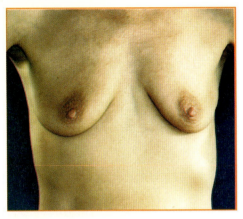

PLATE 7. *(With permission, Michael Cooney/Naturist Society)*

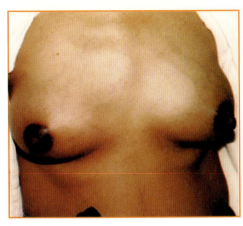

PLATE 8. *(With permission, Kathleen Huggins)*

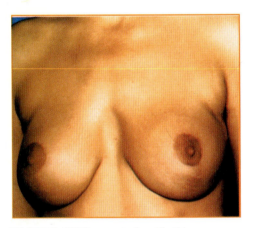

PLATE 9. *(With permission, Kathleen Huggins)*

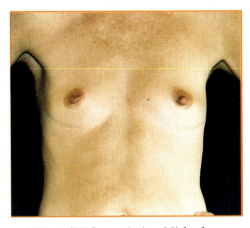

PLATE 10. *(With permission, Michael Cooney/Naturist Society)*

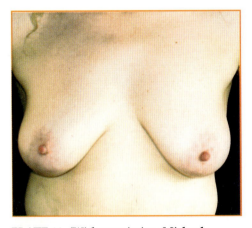

PLATE 11. *(With permission, Michael Cooney/Naturist Society)*

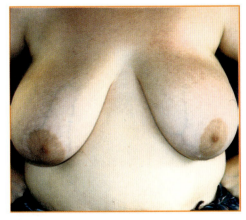

PLATE 12. *(With permission, Michael Cooney/Naturist Society)*

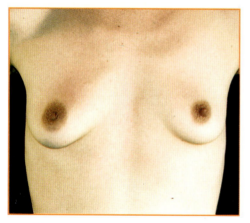

PLATE 13. *(With permission, Michael Cooney/Naturist Society)*

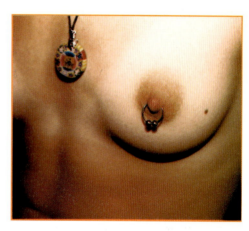

PLATE 14. *(With permission, Kathleen Huggins)*

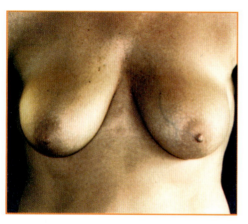

PLATE 15. *(With permission, Michael Cooney/Naturist Society)*

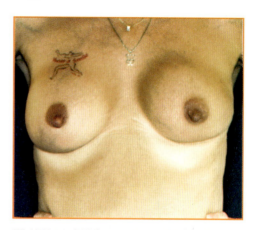

PLATE 16. *(With permission, Michael Cooney/Naturist Society)*

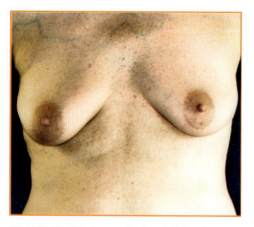

PLATE 17. *(With permission, Michael Cooney/Naturist Society)*

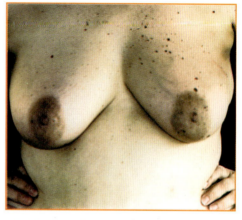

PLATE 18. *(With permission, Michael Cooney/Naturist Society)*

1.2.1 Size

Nipples vary considerably in size and shape. Compare photographs of small nipples (**Plate 19**) with those that are twice as large or larger. In some cases, they are similar to a small coin (U.S. dime). In other cases, the mother's nipples may be considerably larger (**Plate 20**), when compared to a large coin (U.S. quarter).

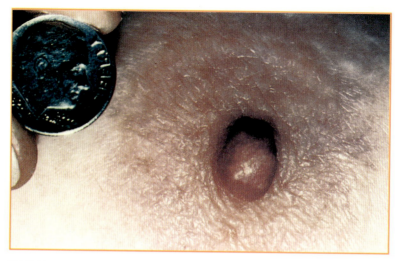

PLATE 19. Nipple in relation to a small coin *(With permission, Kay Hoover)*

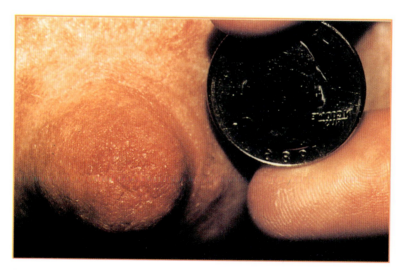

PLATE 20. Nipple in relation to a large coin *(With permission, Kay Hoover)*

Some very large nipples appear to be almost bulbous with the shaft of the nipple narrowing near the areolar tissue **(Plate 21).**

In **Plate 22,** the mother's very large breasts interfered with breastfeeding to the point that the baby was unable to grasp the nipple and breastfeed during the early weeks postpartum. Instead, she used a breast pump with a large-sized flange. In this way, she was able to provide breastmilk for her baby for 5 weeks. By the time the infant weighed 14 pounds, he was able to breastfeed directly. (Note: The tape on the neonate's temple is for a phototherapy mask.)

Some nipples are seated in small areolae; others appear in areolae of varying shapes, and still others appear quite large in relation to the areola. In most cases, the areola is darker than the surrounding breast tissue and is prominent, while a few are very pale in contrast to the color of the skin of the rest of the breast.

Nipple length is also highly variable. A short nipple may be a problem for a newborn to latch onto the breast. Conversely, a long nipple might result in some coughing and choking while the baby learns to accommodate in early breastfeedings. Nipples elongate during the feeding and this elongation is pronounced immediately following a suckling episode.

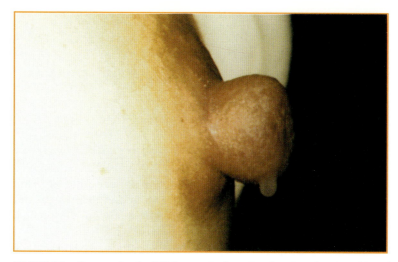

PLATE 21.   Large nipple *(With permission, Carolyn Lawlor-Smith)*

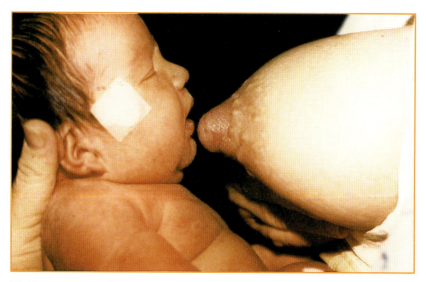

PLATE 22.   Size of newborn mouth in relation to mother's nipple *(With permission, Kathleen Huggins)*

1.2.2 Dimpled nipples

1.2.3 Bifurcated nipples

1.2.4 Folded nipples

Three variations on the usual expectation of nipple eversion are the dimpled nipple (**Plates 23, 24, and 25**), the bifurcated nipple (**Plate 26**) and the folded nipple (**Plate 27**). The woman in Plate 25 bottle-fed her third baby for 2 weeks before seeking help to breastfeed. After using a nipple shield in the early period to bring the baby back to the breast, the dimpling resolved to full eversion. The mother was still breastfeeding 1 year postpartum.

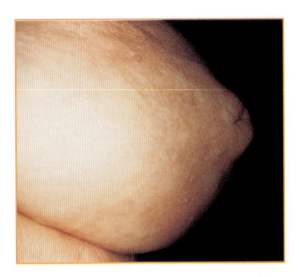

PLATE 23. Side view of dimpled nipple *(With permission, Kathleen G. Auerbach)*

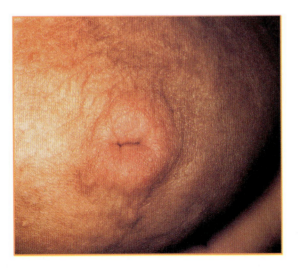

PLATE 24. Front view of dimpled nipple *(With permission, Kathleen G. Auerbach)*

PLATE 25. Dimpled nipple *(With permission, Barbara Wilson-Clay)*

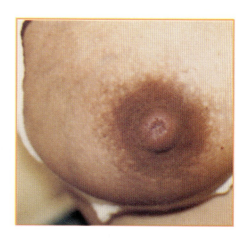

PLATE 26. Bifurcated nipple *(With permission, Robin Egbert)*

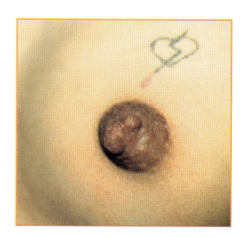

PLATE 27. Folded nipple *(With permission, Kathleen G. Auerbach)*

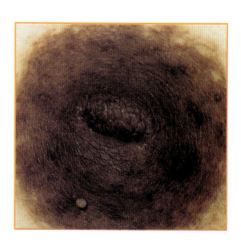

1.2.5 Double nipples

Double nipples may also be present (**Plate 28 and Plate 29**). They need not prevent the baby from breastfeeding.

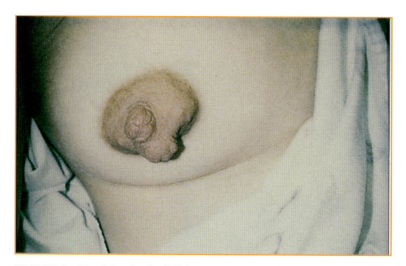

PLATE 28. Double nipple *(With permission, Linda Stewart)*

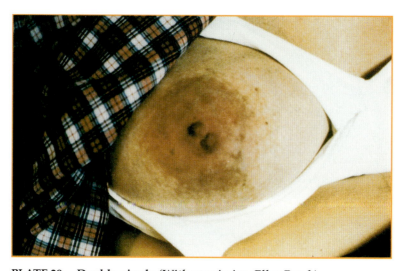

PLATE 29. Double nipple *(With permission, Ellen Petok)*

1.2.6 Inverted nipples

Unlike the variations illustrated earlier, inverted nipples could be a condition that goes beyond a simple variation of normal to a situation that results in difficulty for the baby to grasp and stimulate the breast to release its milk (**Plate 30**). Persons unskilled in assisting in breastfeeding and new mothers may fear that such inversion will always render breastfeeding impossible. This need not be the case. **Plate 31** of the same breast was taken 1 minute after the 2-week-old baby had released the breast.

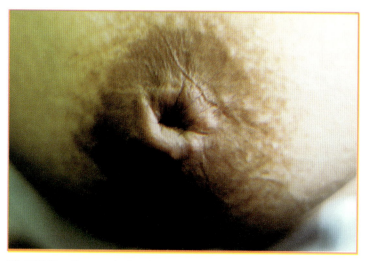

PLATE 30. Inverted nipple *(With permission, Jack Newman)*

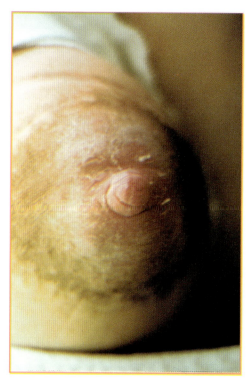

PLATE 31. Inverted nipple immediately
post-suckling by 2-week-old infant *(With
permission, Jack Newman)*

Critical Thinking Activities

The following study questions are designed to stimulate critical thinking and decision-making. Read each question more than once; then look carefully at the color plates. Before answering each question, you might also want to review the corresponding content in the text, *Breastfeeding and Human Lactation, Second Edition.*

These questions may enhance learning in several ways. For example, we encourage readers to use the study questions along with the photographs as case studies where all the possible answers are explored either individually or discussed with colleagues. Teachers can also use these questions in the classroom as a starting point for a lecture. With a computerized overhead projector, the instructor can project the color plates on a screen to students to illustrate specific points.

The authors welcome other suggestions from readers on creative uses of these study questions and the color plates.

1-1.　After answering the questions on page 4 (and checking your answers against the Answer Key found on page 79), note the questions you answered incorrectly.

- What elements led you to your incorrect conclusion(s)?
- What about the photos you identified correctly helped you to make those correct conclusions?
- In what way(s) can you estimate maternal age by visual examination of the breasts/nipples?
- In what way(s) can you estimate maternal parity by visual examination of the breasts/nipples?

1-2.　Look at Plate 19. If you have assisted a woman with very small nipples, what difficulties, if any, did she (or her baby) have with breastfeeding?

- What helping technique(s) were most effective?

1-3.　Plates 20 and 21 present a different potential difficulty from that represented in Plate 19. How often have you encountered a woman whose nipples were too large for her baby's mouth to surround and suckle?

- What helping technique(s) were most effective?
- How did you introduce these suggestions to her?

1-4.　Evaluate the nipples shown in Plates 23 through 31.

- In what way(s) are they similar? Different?
- Which nipple(s) do you feel represent the greatest challenge for a newborn? An infant one month old? A mother breastfeeding for the first time?

- How might the parity of the mother alter the degree of difficulty, if any, which she or her baby might encounter with each type of nipple shown?
- How might the baby's behavior on the breast alter the look of the nipple, the effectiveness of milk transfer, the ease of the suckling experience for the baby?

2

Conditions Affecting the Nipples and/or Breasts

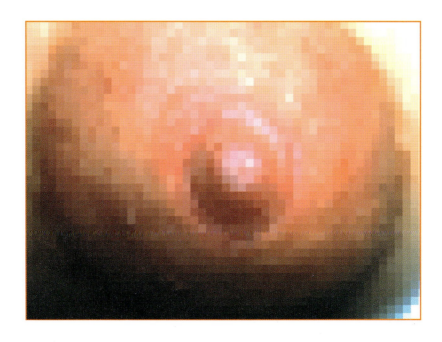

Psoriasis can occur on the nipple **(Plate 32).** A close-up of a patch of psoriasis on a woman's elbow **(Plate 33)** illustrates the characteristic redness interspersed with skin that appears white. A close-up of this condition on the nipple is shown in **Plate 34.**

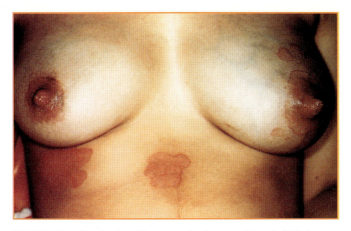

PLATE 32. Psoriasis of breast, nipples, and trunk *(With permission, Chele Marmet/Lactation Institute)*

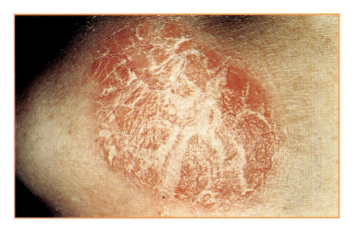

PLATE 33. Psoriasis of the elbow *(With permission, Kay Hoover)*

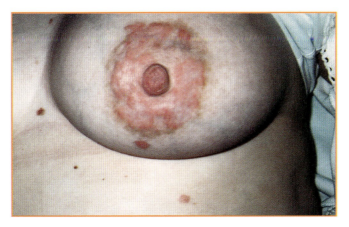

PLATE 34. Close-up of psoriasis on nipple *(With permission, Karen Foard)*

2.2 Poison ivy

Poison ivy can cause characteristic inflammation on any skin surface, including the nipples **(Plate 35).**

2.3 Allergy to antifungal cream

The nipple skin can exhibit an allergic reaction to creams, lotions, and other treatments. **Plate 36** shows a reaction to an antifungal cream.

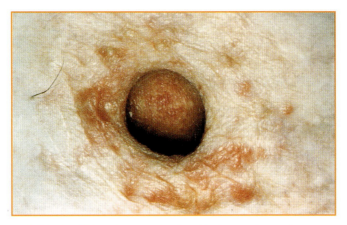

PLATE 35. Poison ivy on nipple *(With permission, Kay Hoover)*

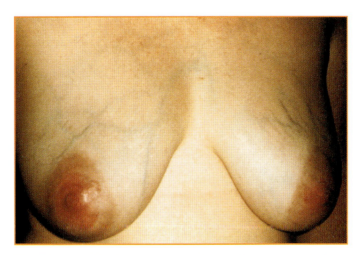

PLATE 36. Allergic reaction to anti-fungal cream on nipples and areola *(With permission, Carolyn Lawlor-Smith)*

2.4 Impetigo

2.5 Dermatitis

2.6 Burns from garlic (home remedy) treatment

Impetigo **(Plate 37)** must be differentiated from candidiasis and dermatitis **(Plate 38),** as all three can present with redness to the skin. However, treatment for one may not resolve other problems. Occasionally treatments for nipple trauma or tenderness cause trauma, as in **Plate 39,** when a mother followed a friend's suggestion to use raw garlic on her tender nipples. The result? Burns where the pieces of fresh garlic touched her skin.

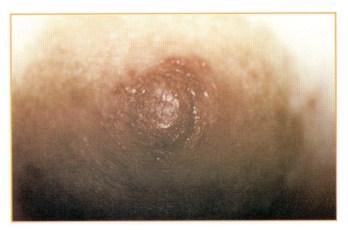

PLATE 37. Impetigo on nipple *(With permission, Kathleen Huggins)*

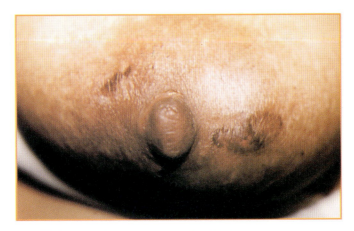

PLATE 38. Dermatitis on nipple *(With permission, Kathleen Huggins)*

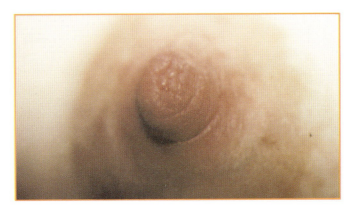

PLATE 39. Garlic burns on areola *(With permission, Kathleen Huggins)*

2.7 Candidiasis of the nipples

Candidiasis appears in a variety of forms on nipple and breast tissue and can be deceptive if the practitioner does not know what to look for. In **Plate 40** and **Plate 41,** the nipple appears to have the same overgrowth (nearly complete to minimal) that is often seen in a baby's mouth (see **Plate 102**). With gentian violet treatment **(Plate 42),** the condition disappears.

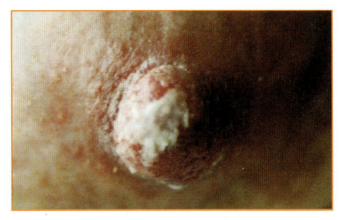

PLATE 40. Candidiasis on nipple *(With permission, Jack Newman)*

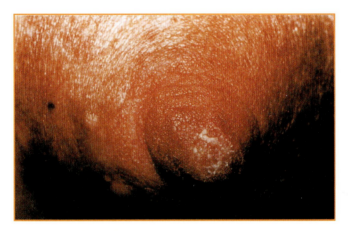

PLATE 41. Candidiasis on nipple *(With permission, Kay Hoover)*

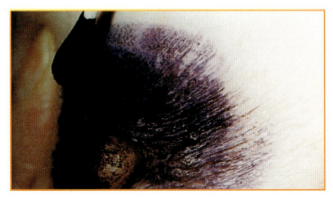

PLATE 42. Gentian violet painting of nipple *(With permission, Kay Hoover)*

In other cases, the nipple may appear with redness or the nipple and areola may have a shiny quality **(Plate 43).** If trauma has been sustained, the site of the wound may exhibit evidence of candidiasis, as seen in **Plate 44.** In this case both some scabbing and yeast overgrowth in and around the nipple crack are visible. The degree of redness with candidiasis is far less noticeable in women with darker skin **(Plate 45)** than in fair-skinned women.

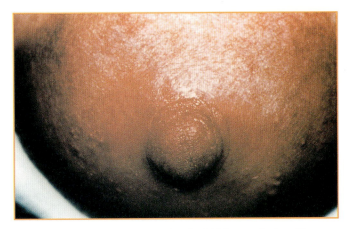

PLATE 43. Candidiasis on nipple *(With permission, Kay Hoover)*

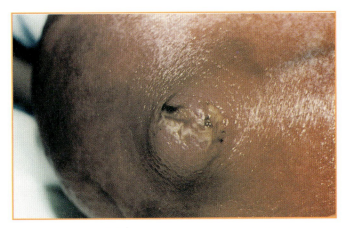

PLATE 44. Candidiasis and trauma on nipple *(With permission, Kay Hoover)*

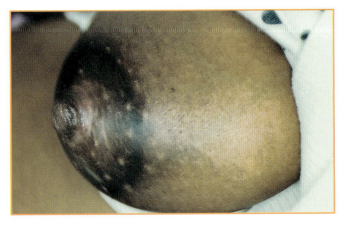

PLATE 45. Candidiasis on nipple *(With permission, Catherine Watson Genna)*

Candidiasis may be accompanied by hypopigmentation of the skin **(Plate 46).** This condition may be more obvious in women with dark skin **(Plate 47)** than in women with pale skin.

Plate 48 shows a mother with tinea versicolor (sometimes called *pityriasis versicolor*), a superficial yeast infection of the trunk. This chronic condition is usually caused by *Pityrosporun orbiculare*. Appropriate treatment includes use of an antifungal cream or ointment.

Candidiasis is not always easily seen on the nipples **(Plate 49).** This mother complained of characteristic burning sensations without visible yeast overgrowth. Treatment for candidiasis resolved her pain. Although the mother's nipples seemed clear, oral candidiasis was identified in the baby's mouth (see **Plate 102**).

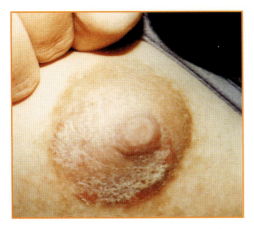

PLATE 46.   Hypopigmentation of areolar skin from candidiasis, Caucasian mother *(With permission, Kay Huggins)*

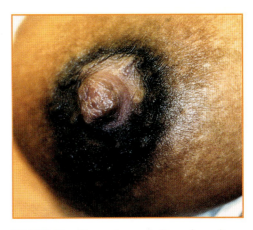

PLATE 47.   Hypopigmentation of areolar skin from candidiasis, African-American mother *(With permission, Catherine Watson Genna)*

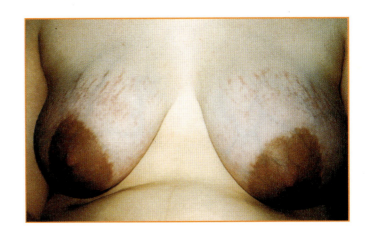

PLATE 48.   Tinea versicolor (petyriasis versicolor) *(With permission, Carolyn Lawlor-Smith)*

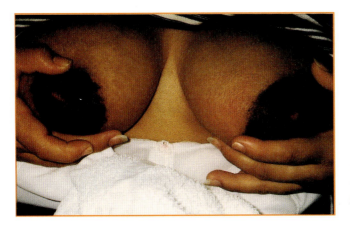

PLATE 49.   No obvious candidiasis *(With permission, Tanna Case-Taylor)*

2.8 Raynaud's phenomenon of the nipple

Raynaud's phenomenon, a blanching and painful "spasm" of the nipple, is poorly understood and may involve only the nipple **(Plate 50)** or the areolar and breast tissue as well. Raynaud's phenomenon can occur with or without a history of the phenomenon in other parts of the body. **Plate 51** shows a primiparous mother with acutely sore nipples from poor latch. The photo was taken within 15 minutes of the baby coming off the breast. The mother reported that blanching began 4 weeks after the start of lactation. Following resolution of the nipple soreness from poor latch, vasospasms ceased within 2 weeks of their first appearance.

Plate 52 and **Plate 53** show the same nipple, first in the midst of a vasospasm and later, after return of blood flow to the area.

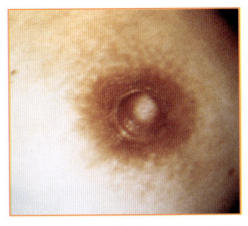

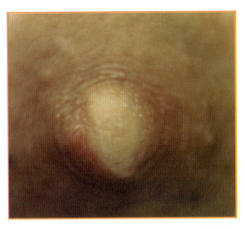

PLATE 50.   Raynaud's phenomenon *(With permission, Carolyn Lawlor-Smith)*

PLATE 51.   Raynaud's phenomenon *(With permission, Jack Newman)*

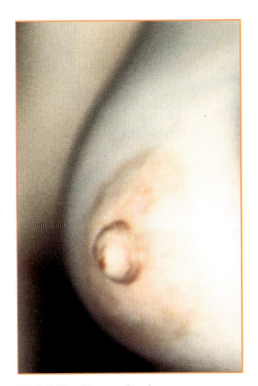

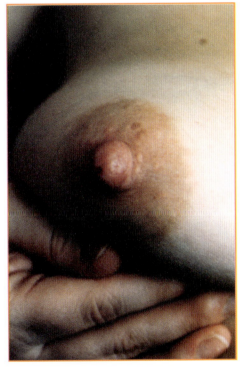

PLATE 52.   Raynaud's phenonemon *(With permission, Lana Matthews)*

PLATE 53.   Same nipple as seen in Plate 52, immediately post-vasospasm episode *(With permission, Lana Matthews)*

2.9 Accessory/supernumerary nipple tissue

Although the norm is two prominent nipples and breasts, nipple and breast tissue can be present from axilla to groin. Accessory nipples may at first be thought to be moles or swollen glands, particularly in nulliparous women. Their presence is often identified when the mother reports swelling during a menstrual cycle or milk production following the baby's birth. **Plate 54** shows a pregnant primigravidous woman whose accessory nipple is not prominent and might be missed if physical examination is cursory.

In some cases **(Plate 55)**, accessory breast tissue may appear as a swelling in the early postpartum period. This tissue may or may not have recognizable nipple tissue.

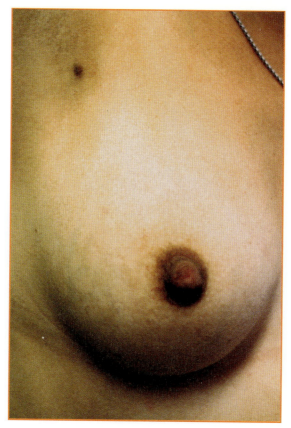

PLATE 54.   Accessory nipple tissue in axilla *(With permission, Jack Newman)*

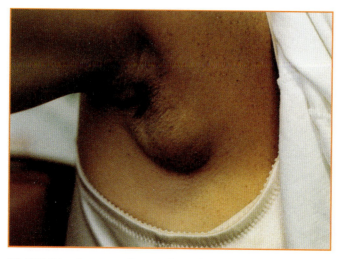

PLATE 55.   Accessory breast tissue in axilla *(With permission, Jack Newman)*

As seen in **Plate 56,** accessory breast tissue may become more prominent as milk production goes into high gear following birth. Sometimes, accessory nipples appear in places other than the axilla **(Plate 57** and **Plate 58).** Note the droplet of milk on the accessory nipple in **Plate 57.**

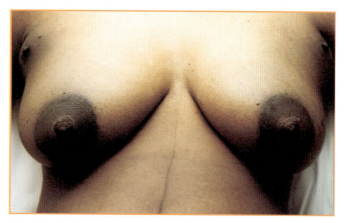

PLATE 56. Accessory breast and nipple tissue, bilaterally *(With permission, Kathleen G. Auerbach)*

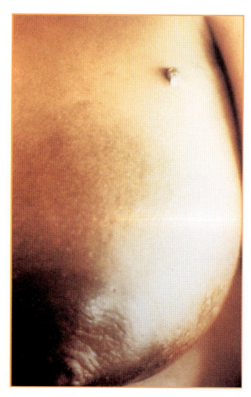

PLATE 57. Accessory nipple tissue near axilla *(With permission, Jack Newman)*

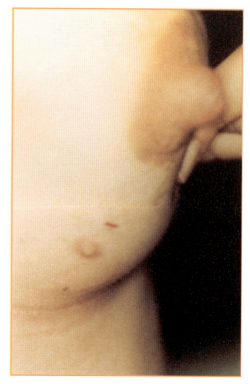

PLATE 58. Accessory nipple tissue on underside of breast *(With permission, Jack Newman)*

2.10 Breast engorgement

Breast engorgement is a common condition of the newly lactating breast **(Plate 59)**. Severe engorgement can result in pain for the mother and difficulty for the baby by impeding the baby's ability to grasp and compress the breast and areolar tissue for milk transfer. Prevention—by early, frequent feedings or expression—is most desirable; however, prompt resolution of the engorgement with culture-specific remedies that include continued breastfeeding through the period of initial excess swelling may also work. In some cases, breast implants or breast reduction surgery may exacerbate the likelihood of engorgement as a result of severing of milk ducts **(Plate 60)**.

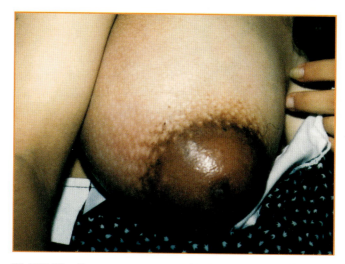

PLATE 59.   Breast engorgement *(With permission, Catherine Watson Genna)*

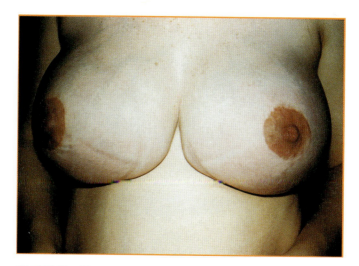

PLATE 60.   Breast engorgement, exacerbated by breast reduction surgery *(With permission, Carolyn Lawlor-Smith)*

2.11 Breast and nipple trauma

Although a folded nipple is usually a normal variation, folding can predispose a mother to the development of tender areas, particularly where the nipple tissue remains wet between feedings. In **Plate 61** (see also **Plate 26**), gently pulling back the nipple folds revealed an area of abrasion that was acutely tender. Treatment was simple: Air drying with a portable hair-dryer after each breastfeeding enhanced healing and felt soothing to the mother. After her first baby had breastfed several months, this mother's folded nipples no longer closed back on themselves! No such abrasion occurred following the birth and early breastfeeding of her second baby.

Poor infant position at the breast sets the stage for breast and nipple trauma. **Plate 62** reveals a wound incurred secondary to sub-optimal positioning. In this case, topical therapy and improved positioning quickly resolved the condition. **Plate 63** reveals a crack on the face of the mother's left nipple caused by suboptimal positioning.

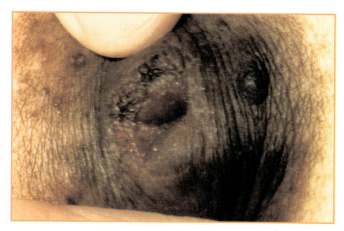

PLATE 61.   Abrasion at site of nipple fold (*With permission,
Kathleen G. Auerbach*)

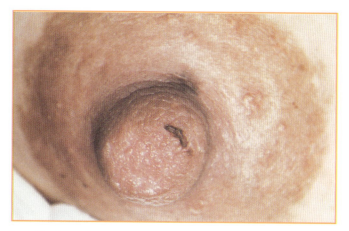

PLATE 62.   Abrasion subsequent to suboptimal positioning
(*With permission, Barbara Wilson-Clay*)

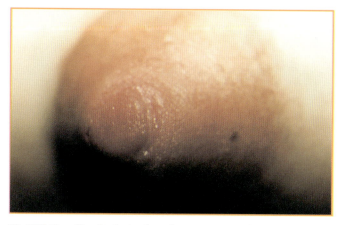

PLATE 63.   Cracked nipple subsequent to suboptimal
positioning (*With permission, Kathleen Huggins*)

Plate 64 shows a severely abraded nipple that took several weeks to heal. Plate 65 illustrates what can happen when a breast pump is not set up appropriately. In this case, the flange insert was not flush with the larger flange. As a result, the skin was repeatedly pinched and trauma occurred.

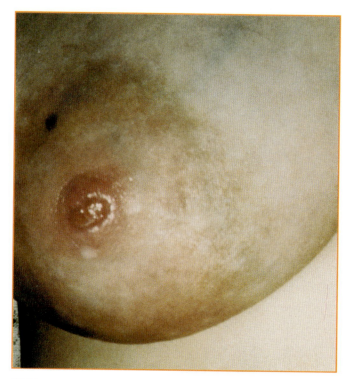

PLATE 64. Severely abraded nipple from suboptimal positioning *(With permission, Catherine Watson Genna)*

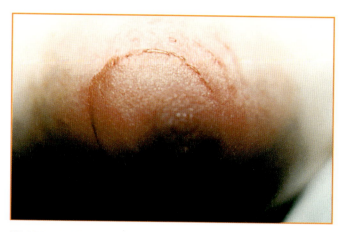

PLATE 65. Trauma from improper configuration of breast pump parts *(With permission, Kathleen Huggins)*

2.12 Mastitis

2.13 Galactocele

Mastitis is an infection characterized by inflammation. It need not preclude continued breastfeeding, and is more rapidly resolved when breastfeeding continues on the affected side. Following such infection, the mother will likely have a tender area, around which her skin assumes a redder aspect **(Plate 66).** Her milk supply may be temporarily diminished in the affected breast.

Plate 67 shows a mother's breast in which a galactocele (a cyst filled with milk) developed. In this case, 90 ml of milk was obtained the first time the galactocele was drained. After several additional drainings, the galactocele resolved and breastfeeding continued without difficulty.

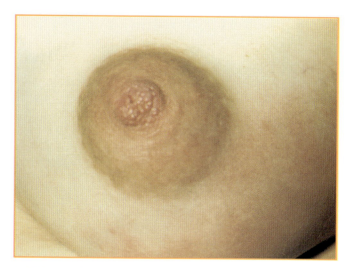

PLATE 66.   Mastitis *(With permission, Kathleen G. Auerbach)*

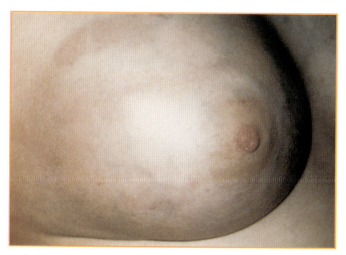

PLATE 67.   Galactocele *(With permission, Carolyn Lawlor-Smith)*

Abscess of the breast frequently can be avoided if mastitis is managed appropriately and early. However, abscess can still occur and is a serious health problem that should be treated vigorously with antibiotics under the supervision of a physician.

In **Plate 68,** a primiparous mother approximately 4 weeks postpartum presented with what appeared to be unresolved mastitis in her right breast. Note the raised area in the upper inner aspect at about the 2 o'clock position. This abscess was aspirated, followed by incision and drainage for complete resolution of the problem. In **Plate 69,** the mother's abscess was drained under local anesthesia and she continued breastfeeding on the affected side.

In some cases, the abscess will spontaneously erupt, as seen in **Plate 70.** Visible in the abscess wound is the mother's breast implant. Although not implicated in the development of the abscess, this mother had her implants removed after treatment, which was complicated by their presence.

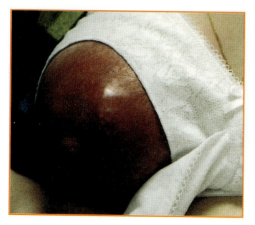

PLATE 68. Breast abscess *(With permission, Jack Newman)*

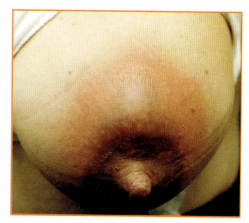

PLATE 69. Breast abscess *(With permission, Jack Newman)*

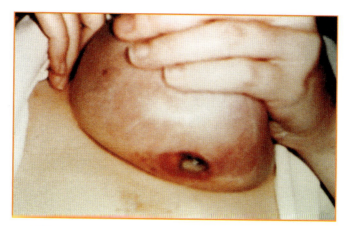

PLATE 70. Spontaneously ruptured breast abscess *(With permission, Ellen Petok)*

Although rare, an abscess can occur more than once in the same breast. In **Plate 71,** the first abscess lies superior to the more recent one with pus still draining from the incision site. The current abscess appears closer to the nipple and slightly exterior to the first. **Plate 72** illustrates aspiration of a breast abscess in the lower outer quadrant of the left breast in a mother 6 weeks postpartum. Note that milk at the nipple pores appears normal.

Plate 73 shows the outcome of surgical incision and draining of an abscess before healing is completed. The mother continued breast-feeding.

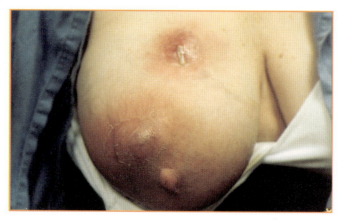

PLATE 71. Two abscesses in the same breast *(With permission, Jack Newman)*

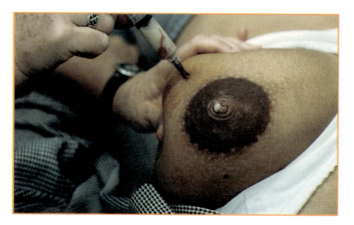

PLATE 72. Aspiration of breast abscess *(With permission, Jack Newman)*

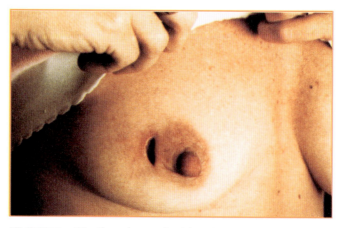

PLATE 73. Healing abscess incision *(With permission, Ellen Petok)*

2.15 Scarring of the breast

Any breast surgery can cause scarring. In some cases, scars are difficult to see; in other cases, keloidal tissue will make it obvious (see **Plate 81**). The mother in Plate 74 had an incision at the external areolar margin on her right breast between the 9 and 12 o'clock positions. Surgery may have been done to remove a benign cyst or to insert a breast implant. Whatever the reason, scarring at this site should serve as a marker for potential problems with milk production and transfer. Scarring at the areolar margin usually means that milk ducts and nerves have been severed, thus reducing both nipple ennervation and milk transfer through the affected ducts.

Occasionally, scarring may result from cosmetic additions, as following the placement of a nipple ring **(Plate 14)**. Whether the insertion of the ring will negatively affect breastfeeding can only be determined after the mother puts her baby to breast. This is more easily accomplished after removing the ring!

Plate 75 shows a pattern of scarring characteristic of recently conducted breast reduction surgery. Note that the surgical procedure involves the nipple, with periareolar scarring from complete removal of the nipple and repositioning on the smaller breast. Surgery may result in altered or no sensation following nipple stimulation.

In some cases, periareolar scarring from breast implants is difficult to see **(Plate 76)** and may only be acknowledged when the mother's initial complaint is some other problem, such as nipple trauma caused by the baby's strenuous efforts to obtain milk.

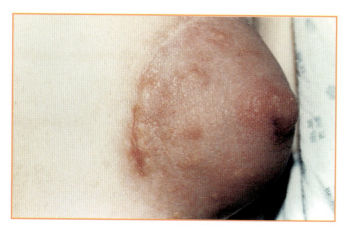

PLATE 74.   Areolar scar *(With permission, Kay Hoover)*

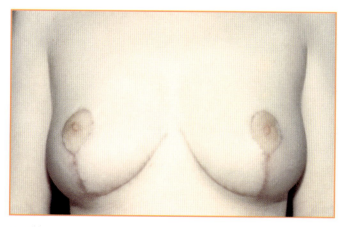

PLATE 75.   Scarring from breast reduction surgery *(With permission, Diana West)*

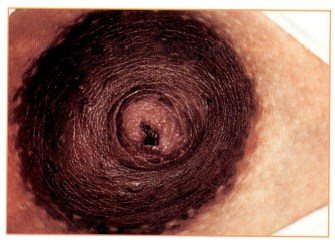

PLATE 76.   Periareolar scarring and positional trauma *(With permission, Barbara Wilson-Clay)*

Reduction mammoplasty may leave scars on the breast at or near the areola, or elsewhere. As seen in **Plate 77,** a lateral wedge technique was used. Although this woman had concerns about her milk production, the baby gained well without supplements.

Plate 78 shows both visible scarring (upper aspect of the left breast) and the absence of the right nipple. This woman was unable to breastfeed following surgical treatment for breast lumps at age 19 and subsequent post-operative infection. Additional surgery was attempted to treat the infection, at which time the right nipple was severely damaged.

Plate 79 shows a scar from an incision to drain an abscess that occurred 2 years previously. This type of lateral incision is likely to interfere with subsequent breastfeeding because several milk ducts have been severed. At the time this picture was taken, the pregnant mother asked about her ability to breastfeed her expected baby.

Plate 80 shows a 19-year-old woman with Poland syndrome, a congenital condition in which the pectoralis major muscle and one breast are absent. Also seen are marks showing the incision site for insertion of a breast implant. This woman will be able to breastfeed only from the normally developed breast.

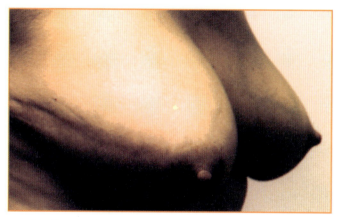

PLATE 77. Reduction mammoplasty scar, wedge technique *(With permission, Ellen Petok)*

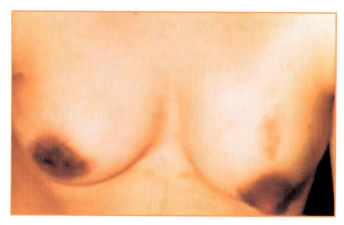

PLATE 78. Scarring above left breast and destruction of right nipple *(With permission, Kathleen Huggins)*

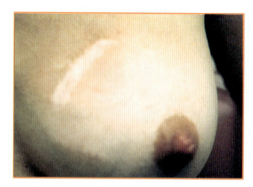

PLATE 79. Healed abscess incision scar *(With permission, Jack Newman)*

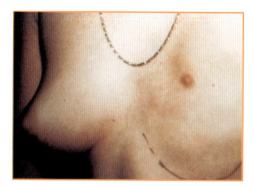

PLATE 80. Poland syndrome with marks showing incision for breast implant *(With permission, Carolyn Lawlor-Smith)*

Plate 81 shows a young mother who was badly burned in a house fire when she was a child. She sustained marked scarring over her entire trunk area. Cosmetic surgery performed years after the fire created nipple tissue in an effort to render her developing breasts a more normal appearance.

Plate 82 reveals telltale scars in the lower right quadrant and a suggestion of at least one intact nipple pore near the center of the nipple. The presence of this pore was confirmed while observing the mother pumping her breast. Unlike the other nipple, which only dripped milk **(Plate 83),** the intact pore streamed milk with minimal stimulation. Although her first child breastfed with initial assistance from a feeding tube device to assure adequate milk transfer, within 1 month the baby needed no supplements, nor did the mother's second infant. The message from this case (and others included in this collection of photographs) is clear: form (the look of the mother's breasts) need not always predict function (their ability to respond to appropriate stimulation).

The woman pictured in **Plate 84** is breastfeeding after experiencing a unilateral mastectomy following a diagnosis of breast cancer.

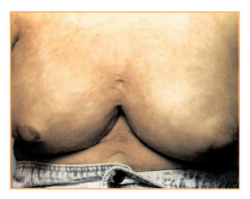

PLATE 81.   Burn scars *(With permission, Kathleen G. Auerbach)*

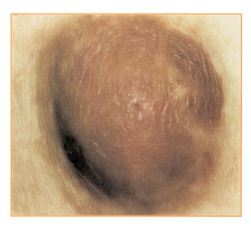

PLATE 82.   Left nipple reconstruction, one intact nipple pore *(With permission, Kathleen G. Auerbach)*

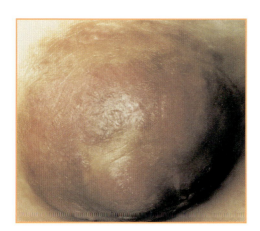

PLATE 83.   Right nipple reconstruction *(With permission, Kathleen G. Auerbach)*

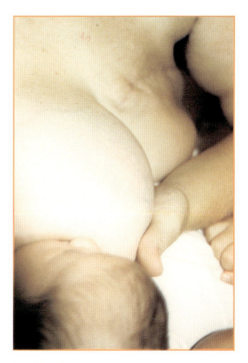

PLATE 84.   Left mastectomy scar *(With permission, Barbara Wilson-Clay)*

2.16 Breast asymmetry and hypoplasia

Asymmetry of the breasts may be part of normal variation that does not usually affect lactation. The woman in **Plate 85** did not breastfeed her child; the woman in **Plate 86** did, with no reported difficulties.

In other cases, asymmetry appears to be associated with reduced capacity to produce milk. The question arises: Are certain breast structures associated with primary breast insufficiency? For example, the mother in **Plate 87** produced less milk from her smaller breast. This difference in production, however, did not prevent her from maintaining a breastfeeding relationship with her infant. In some cases, an initial low or inadequate milk supply may be transient, occurring early in the lactational process and resolving spontaneously over time as a result of frequent, effective suckling by the baby. In other cases, supplementation is necessary.

Breast hypoplasia is incomplete development of the breasts. This condition can result in seriously impaired milk production **(Plate 88).** This mother had to supplement in order to assure appropriate infant growth. In addition to the shape and size of her breasts, note the shape of her nipples and the wide spacing between her breasts.

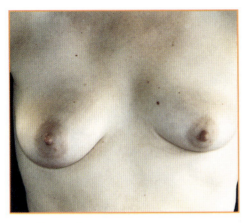

PLATE 85. Breast asymmetry *(With permission, Michael Cooney/Naturist Society)*

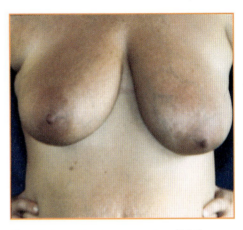

PLATE 86. Breast asymmetry *(With permission, Michael Cooney/Naturist Society)*

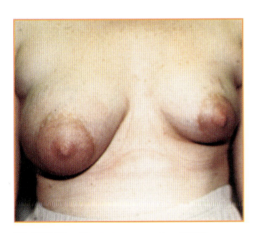

PLATE 87. Breast asymmetry *(With permission, Ellen Petok)*

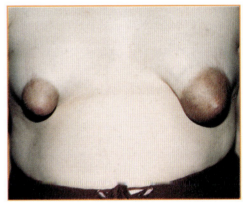

PLATE 88. Breast hypoplasia *(With permission, Ellen Petok)*

Plate 89 shows a mother with minimal breast tissue whose milk production was negligible in the first 10 days postpartum. However, she progressed to full production with continued frequent stimulation, in contrast to the other women in this group who made little or no milk.

The mother in Plate 90 has breasts that superficially appear to be normal. However, milk production—even with frequent stimulation—was insufficient to nourish her infant without supplementation. Note the wide space between her breasts.

In Plate 91, the right nipple appears to sit on a bulbous areola with minimal breast tissue behind it. This mother's baby experienced very slow weight gain in the first month of breastfeeding and then rapid catch-up growth without supplementation thereafter. The left breast (not pictured) was markedly larger than the right breast with the same appearance of nipple and areola.

In Plate 92, the mother's nipple and areolar tissue appears abnormally enlarged, giving an impression of a "dome" crowning the breast.

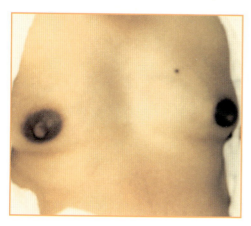

PLATE 89.   Minimal breast tissue; delayed milk production *(With permission, Kathleen Huggins)*

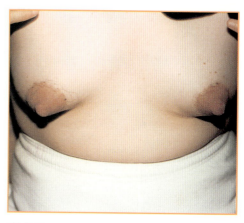

PLATE 90.   Widely spaced breasts; milk insufficiency *(With permission, Kathleen Huggins)*

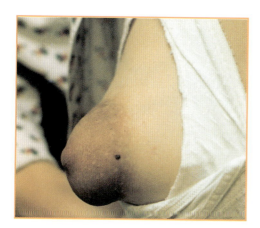

PLATE 91.   Bulbous areola *(With permission, Jack Newman)*

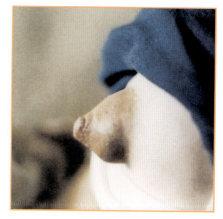

PLATE 92.   Abnormally enlarged, "domed" areola *(With permission, Ellen Petok)*

Critical Thinking Activities

The following study questions are designed to stimulate critical thinking and decision-making. Read each question more than once; then look carefully at the color plates. Before answering each question, you might also want to review the corresponding content in the text, *Breastfeeding and Human Lactation, Second Edition.*

2-1. Describe psoriasis (see Plates 32-34).

■ How does it differ in appearance by where it occurs on the body?
■ If you have assisted a mother who had psoriasis, what technique(s) were most effective?

2-2. Examine the "look" of the dermatologic conditions shown in Plates 35 through 39.

■ In what way(s) if any, are they alike (or different) in . . .

appearance?
likelihood of pain?
likelihood of chronicity of the condition?
acuity of the condition?
effect on the mother's breastfeeding plan?
ability of the baby to continue breastfeeding?
need for medication to resolve the problem?

2-3. Examine Plates 40 through 47, and Plate 49.

■ Which plate characterizes most closely the women you have seen with this condition?
■ In what way(s) does the variation in presentation render assessment and diagnosis

more difficult than the other dermatologic conditions that can occur on breasts/nipples?
less difficult than the other dermatologic conditions that can occur on breasts/nipples?

■ What signs and symptoms (in mother, in baby) do you believe are most indicative of the presence of candidiasis as shown in Plate 49?

2-4. How is Raynaud's phenomenon different from hypopigmentation secondary to candidiasis? (see Plates 50 through 53)

■ What symptoms have you found to be most suggestive of Raynaud's phenomenon?
■ How frequent (in your practice) is Raynaud's phenomenon?
■ How might its frequency of occurrence relate to your consideration of it as a problem a mother presents when her primary complaint is pain?

Critical Thinking Activities

2-5. Examine Plates 54 through 58. Where on a mother's body have you identified accessory breast or nipple tissue?

- In what way(s) does the presence of milk in accessory breast/nipple tissue cause concern?
- How might you assist a mother with accessory breast/nipple tissue. Consider the placement of such tissue in your response.

2-6. Breast engorgement is illustrated in Plates 59 and 60.

- How might the engorgement illustrated affect the mother's baby's experience with early breastfeeding?
- In what way(s) might her breast surgery have made breast engorgement . . .

more likely to occur?
more likely to take longer to resolve?
more difficult for the baby to breastfeed?

2-7. Nipple trauma can occur as a result of numerous situations (see Plates 61 through 65).

- In what way(s) were these different examples of nipple trauma similarly caused?
- How might you help a mother resolve each of these injuries?
- How might you help a mother reduce the likelihood of experiencing each of these injuries?

2-8. Distinguish between mastitis and galactocele (see Plates 66 and 67).

- In what way(s) might a mother with each of these conditions be at risk for abscess?
- What technique(s) would you recommend to resolve . . .

mastitis?
galactocele?

2-9. Examine Plates 68 through 73.

- What do these photos tell you about this condition?
- In what way(s) are these plates illustrative of abscess cases you have been asked to help resolve?
- What treatment(s) would you recommend to help a mother resolve this condition?
- How would you respond to a woman who concludes that she should stop breastfeeding after learning that her abscess requires incision and drainage?

2-10. Examine Plates 75 through 79, 81 through 84.

- List the causes of scarring on the breast.
- Which of these causes are likely to interfere with continued breast-feeding?
- Which of these causes are not likely to interfere with continued breastfeeding?
- Which of these causes represent the greatest impact on adequate milk transfer?
- What management recommendations would you suggest for each reason for breast scarring that . . .

  you mentioned above?
  as illustrated in Plates 75 through 79, 81 through 84.

- Of the women you have assisted who presented with breast scarring, how many continue to breastfeed?
- What means of assistance did you provide the women represented in your answer that was most effective?

2-11. Examine Plate 80. What is Poland syndrome?

- How might you identify the existence of Poland syndrome if your first encounter with a woman occurs several hours following the birth of her first child?
- If asked by a woman with this syndrome about her likelihood of breastfeeding, what would you tell her?

2-12. Examine Plates 85 through 90.

- What similarities and differences do you observe?
- Which of these photos suggest possible insufficient milk syndrome?
- What management recommendation(s) would you offer in the case of actual milk insufficiency?
- Under what circumstance(s), if any, would you recommend against continued breastfeeding? Explain your answer.

2-13. Review Plates 91 and 92.

- What about these areolar shapes suggest:

  (in)adequacy of milk production?
  infant difficulty obtaining sufficient milk?

- How might these areolar shapes be related to breast hypoplasia?

3

Infant Conditions

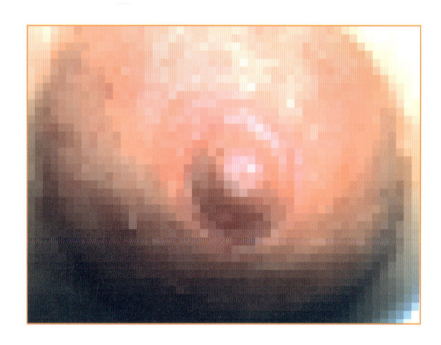

3.1 Buccal fat pads in a normal infant

Term infants have buccal fat pads on the interior side of each cheek that stabilize positioning of anything drawn into or inserted into the infant's mouth, such as a breast **(Plate 93).** These fat pads gradually disappear through the first year of life.

3.2 Hemangioma of the tongue

Hemangioma, a benign vascular tumor, of the tongue is a rare congenital anomaly **(Plate 94).** Shortly after birth, this baby latched and breastfed well. However, an untreated hemangioma may interfere with later ability to feed by causing increasing obstruction.

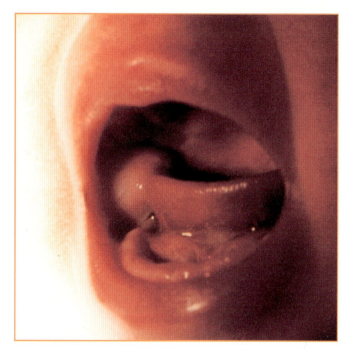

PLATE 93. Buccal fat pads in newborn *(With permission, Jan Riordan)*

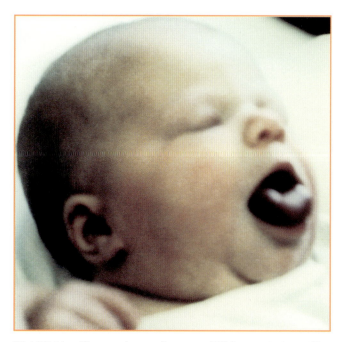

PLATE 94. Hemangioma of tongue *(With permission, Ellen Petok)*

3.3 Cleft of the lip and/or palate

Clefts can occur in the neonate's lip, in the palate, or both. The baby in **Plate 95** was able to breastfeed well when the mother assisted in securing more complete sealing of the lip at the site of the cleft.

The baby in **Plate 96** and **Plate 97** has a unilateral cleft of the lip and hard palate. The baby in **Plate 98** was able to breastfeed shortly after her cleft lip was repaired at 10 weeks. This baby was fed at breast with the assistance of a tube feeding device. Following repair of the palate, she continued to breastfeed for 2 years.

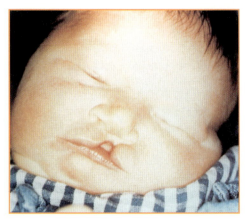

PLATE 95. Unilateral cleft of lip *(With permission, Barbara Wilson-Clay*

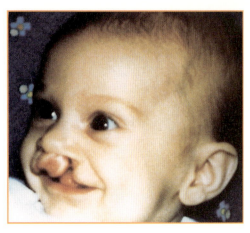

PLATE 96. Unilateral cleft of lip *(With permission, Ellen Petok)*

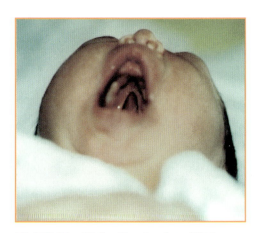

PLATE 97. Cleft of hard palate *(With permission, Ellen Petok)*

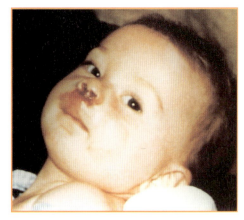

PLATE 98. Repaired cleft of lip *(With permission, Ellen Petok)*

3.4 Ankyloglossia (tongue-tie)

Ankyloglossia (tongue-tie) is a tethering of the tongue so that it cannot extend over the lower gum and thus interferes with suckling at the breast. In some cases, tongue-tie is obvious **(Plate 99),** often demonstrating a characteristic heart shape or notch at the site of the tether when the baby attempts to lift the tongue. In other cases, the condition may not be discovered until the mother complains of chronic nipple soreness, the infant has difficulty with breastfeeding (including failure to thrive) and/or the baby's mouth is assessed **(Plate 100).** In **Plate 101,** the same baby's tongue is untethered following simple clipping of the frenulum (frenotomy). Both parents of this infant had the condition as children.

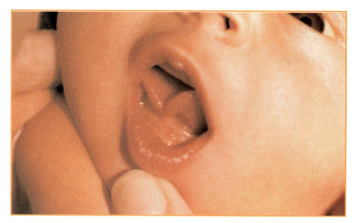

PLATE 99. Ankyloglossia *(With permission, Kathleen Huggins)*

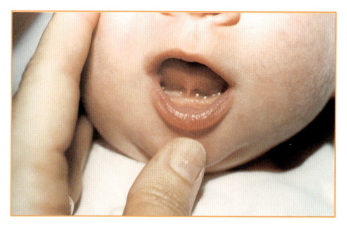

PLATE 100. Ankyloglossia *(With permission, Barbara Wilson-Clay)*

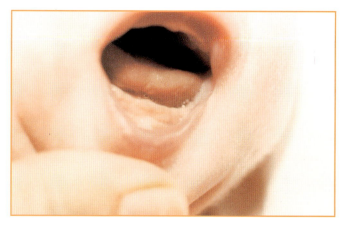

PLATE 101. Infant tongue following frenotomy *(With permission, Barbara Wilson-Clay)*

3.5 Thrush in the infant

3.5.1 Oral

3.5.2 Diaper area

White growth (oral thrush) in the baby's mouth, on or behind the tongue, and on the buccal pads or gums is diagnostic evidence of candidiasis **(Plate 102)**. **Plate 103** and **Plate 104** show diaper area candidiasis in a female and male infant, respectively. This overt evidence of thrush is not always present even when the infant has candidiasis.

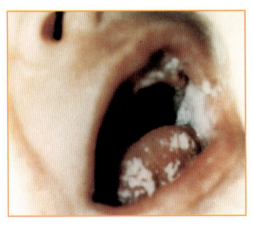

PLATE 102. Oral thrush *(With permission, Kay Hoover)*

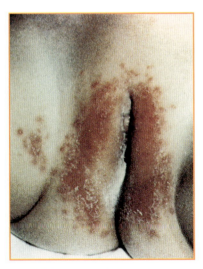

PLATE 103. Candidiasis in diaper area, female infant *(With permission, Kay Hoover)*

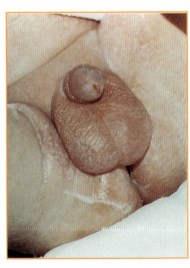

PLATE 104. Candidiasis in diaper area, male infant *(With permission, Kay Hoover)*

The following study questions are designed to stimulate critical thinking and decision-making. Read each question more than once; then look carefully at the color plates. Before answering each question, you might also want to review the corresponding content in the text, *Breastfeeding and Human Lactation, Second Edition.*

3-1.   Examine Plate 93.

   ■ How would you explain to a mother the function of buccal fat pads . . .

      in a fullterm infant?
      if her baby is born prematurely?

3-2.   How might hemangioma of the tongue (Plate 94) interfere with breast-feeding?

3-3.   Examine Plates 95 through 98.

   ■ Which of these infants most closely represents situations in which you have assisted a mother with a baby with cleft lip/palate?
   ■ In what way(s) might bilateral cleft lip/palate represent greater difficulty with breastfeeding?
   ■ What would you tell a mother who is concerned about breastfeeding a baby with this congenital defect?

3-4.   Examine Plates 99 through 101.

   ■ Under what circumstances would you recommend frenotomy to resolve the baby's tongue-tie?
   ■ When would you not make this recommendation?
   ■ Of the breastfeeding couples you have assisted, what signs/symptoms suggested ankyloglossia as the presenting problem?

3-3.   Examine Plates 102 through 104.

   ■ What signs/symptoms additional to visible yeast overgrowth might these infants exhibit?
   ■ How would you treat an infant with this condition?
   ■ What treatment recommendations would you offer the mothers of these babies . . .

      for herself?
      for other family members?

Answer key

Answer key to the questions appearing on page 3.

1. 11, 12, 13, 14, 16
2. 6
3. 14
4. 2
5. 3
6. 16
7. 9
8. 8
9. 7

INDEX

A

Abrasions
    nipple, 42, **43 (Plates 61 and 62),** 44,
        45 (Plate 64)
Abscess 48, **49 (Plates 68 and 70),** 50, **51**
    (Plates 71–73)
    scarring, 54, **55 (Plate 79)**
Accessory tissue
    breast 36, **37 (Plate 55),** 38, **39 (Plate**
        56)
    nipple, 36, **37 (Plates 54 and 55)**
Antifungal cream
    allergy to, 24, **25 (Plate 35)**
Ankyloglossia (tongue-tie), 72, **73**
    (Plates 99–101)
Areolae
    bulbous, 60, **61 (Plate 91)**
    enlarged or "dome", 60, **61 (Plate**
        92)
    scarring, 52, **53 (Plate 74)**
    shiny quality, 30, **31 (Plate 43)**
Aspiration
    of breast abscess, 50, **51 (Plate 72)**
Asymmetry
    of breasts, 58, **59 (Plates 85–87),** 60,
        61 (Plates 89–92)

B

Babies. *see* infant conditions
Blanching, 34, **35 (Plates 50 and 51)**

Breast(s)
    accessory, 36, **37 (Plate 55),** 38, **39**
        (Plate 56)
    asymmetry, 58, **59 (Plates 85–87),** 60,
        61 (Plates 89–92)
    cyst, milk-filled, 46, **47 (Plate 67)**
    engorgement, 40, **41 (Plates 59 and**
        60)
    hypoplasia, 58, **59 (Plate 88),** 60, **61**
        (Plate 90)
    implants, 40, 48, **49 (Plate 70)**
        scarring from, 52, **53 (Plate 76)**
    pumps, improper configuration, 44,
        45 (Plate 65)
    reduction surgery 40, **41 (Plate 60)**
        scarring pattern, 52, **53 (Plate 75)**
Buccal fat pads, 68, **69 (Plate 93)**
Burns
    scarring from, 56, **57 (Plate 81)**

C

Candidiasis
    in baby's mouth, 28, 32, **75 (Plate 102)**
    of nipples, 28, **29 (Plates 40 and 41),**
        30, **31 (Plates 43–45),** 32, **33**
        (Plates 46–49)
    oral, 32, 74, **75 (Plate 102)**
Cleft
    of the lip and/or palate, 70, **71**
        (Plates 95–98)
Critical Thinking Activities, 19, 63, 77

Cyst
    milk-filled, 46, **47 (Plate 67)**

D

Dermatitis, 26, **27 (Plate 38)**

E

Engorgement
    breast, 40, **41 (Plates 59 and 60)**
Eversion
    nipple, 12

F

Form, 4, 56
Frenotomy, 72, **73 (Plate 101)**
Function and form, 4, 56

G

Galactocele
    46, **47 (Plate 67)**

H

Hemangioma
    of tongue, 68, **69 (Plate 94)**
Hypopigmentation, 32, **33 (Plate 46)**
Hypoplasia, 58, **59 (Plate 88),** 60, **61
    (Plate 90)**

I

Impetigo, 26, **27 (Plate 37)**
Infant conditions
    ankyloglossia, 72, **73 (Plates 99–101)**
    buccal fat pads, 68, **69 (Plate 93)**
    cleft of lip and/or palate, 70, **71
        (Plates 95–98)**
    hemangioma, of tongue, 68, **69
        (Plate 94)**
    thrush, oral, 74, **75 (Plates 102–104)**
    tongue-tie, 72, **73 (Plates 99-100)**

M

Mastectomy, 56, **57 (Plate 84)**
Mastitis, 46, **47 (Plate 66),** 48

N

Nipple
    abrasions, 42, **43 (Plates 61 and 62),**
        44, **45 (Plate 64)**

accessory, 36, **37 (Plates 54 and 55)**
bifurcated, 12, **13 (Plate 26)**
blanching, 34, **35 (Plates 50 and 51)**
candidiasis on, 32, **33 (Plate 49)**
dimpled, 12, **13 (Plates 23–25)**
double, 14, **15 (Plates 28 and 29)**
folded, 12, **13 (Plate 27),** 42, **43 (Plate
    61)**
hypopigmentation of, 32, **33 (Plate
    46)**
infections, yeast, 32, **33 (Plate 48)**
inverted, 16, **17 (Plates 30 and 31)**
length, 10
Raynaud's phenomenon of, 34, **35
    (Plates 50-53)**
redness, 30, **31 (Plate 43)**
ring, **7 (Plate 14),** 52
scarring. *see* scarring of the breast
shiny quality of, 30, **31 (Plate 43)**
size of, 8, **9, (Plates 19 and 20),** 10, **11
    (Plates 21 and 22)**
tissue, supernumerary, 36, **37 (Plates
    54 and 55)**
trauma to, 30, **31 (Plate 44)**

P

Pityriasis versicolor, 32, **33 (Plate 48)**
Pityrosproum orbiculare, 32, **33 (Plate 48)**
Poison ivy, 24, **25 (Plate 35)**
Poland syndrome, 54, **55 (Plate 80)**
Positioning suboptimal, 42, **43 (Plates 62
    and 63),** 44, **45 (Plate 64)**

R

Raynaud's phenomenon, 34, **35 (Plates
    50–53)**

S

Scarring
    of breasts, 52, **53 (Plates 74–76),** 54,
        55 (Plates 77–80), 56, **57 (Plates
        81–84)**
Self-test, 4–7
    answers, 77
Surgery
    scarring from, 52, **53 (Plate 75),** 54,
        55 (Plates 77 and 78), 56, **57
        (Plates 81 and 84)**

see also breast implants; breast reduction surgery

T

Thrush
    in infant, 74 **(Plates 102–104)**
    oral, 74, **75 (Plates 102-104)**
Tinea versicolor, 32, **33 (Plate 48)**
Tongue
    hemangioma, 68, **69 (Plate 94)**
    -tie, 72, **73 (Plates 99–101)**
Trauma
    to breasts and nipples, 42, **43 (Plates 61–63),** 44, **45 (Plates 64 and 65)**
    to nipples, 30, **31 (Plate 44)**

Treatment
    garlic (home remedy), 26, **27 (Plate 39)**
    gentian violet, 28, **29 (Plate 42)**

V

Vasospasm, 34, **35 (Plates 52 and 53)**

Y

Yeast
    infection, 32, **33 (Plate 48)**